T0198769

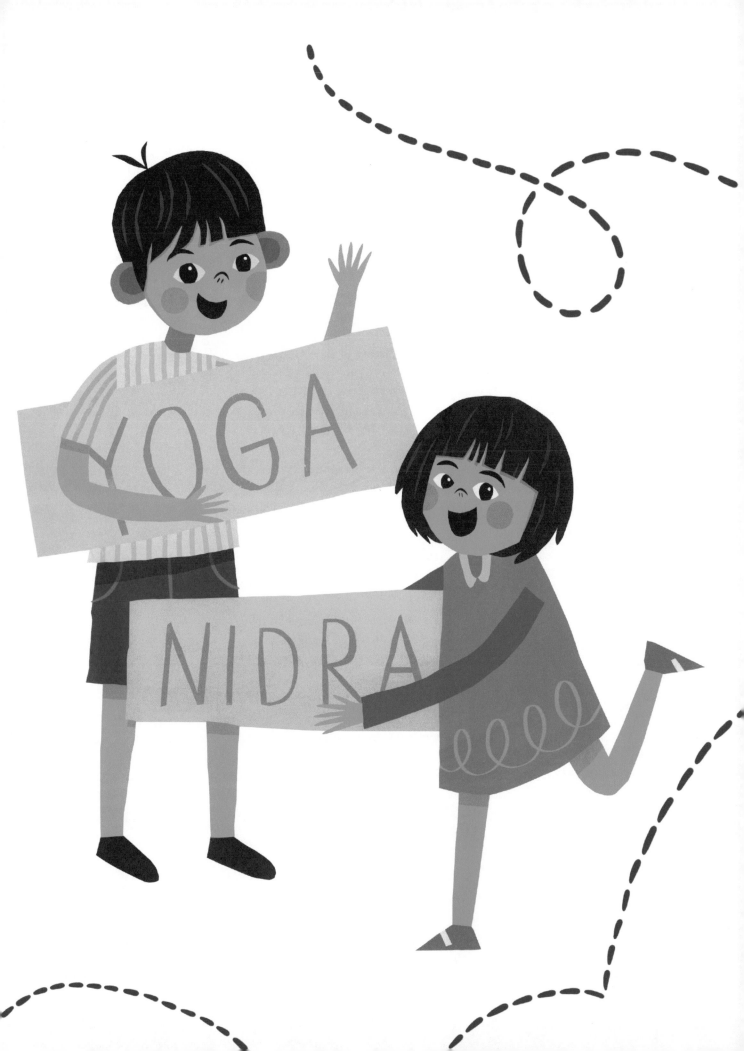

Balboa Press books may be ordered through booksellers or by contacting:

Balboa Press
A Division of Hay House
1663 Liberty Drive
Bloomington, IN 47403
www.balboapress.com
844-682-1282

ISBN: 978-1-9822-7569-3 (sc)
ISBN: 978-1-9822-7571-6 (hc)
ISBN: 978-1-9822-7570-9 (e)

Library of Congress Control Number: 2021920883

Print information available on the last page.

Balboa Press rev. date: 09/21/2023

BALBOA.PRESS
A DIVISION OF HAY HOUSE

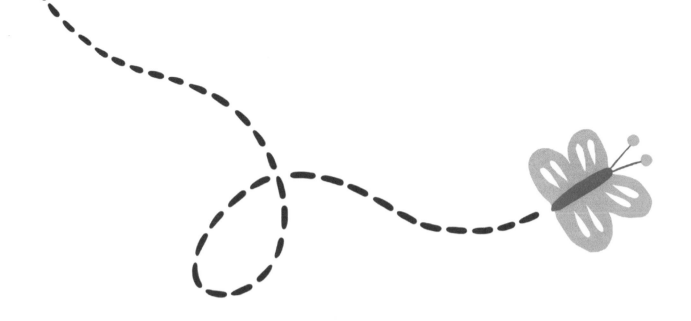

This book is dedicated to

Young Yogis everywhere.
Rahul and Ria, who inspired the
illustrated characters.

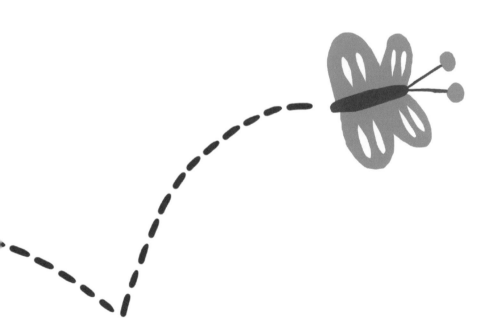

Let's get ready to practice **Yoga Nidra.**

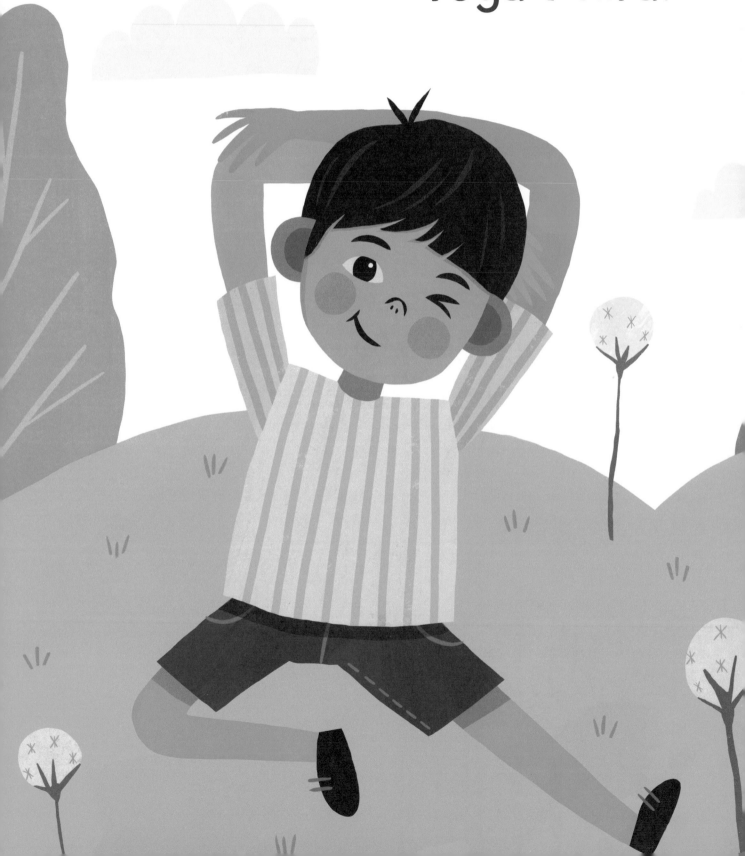

Yoga Nidra.
A journey of the **body**.
A journey of the **breath**.
A journey.

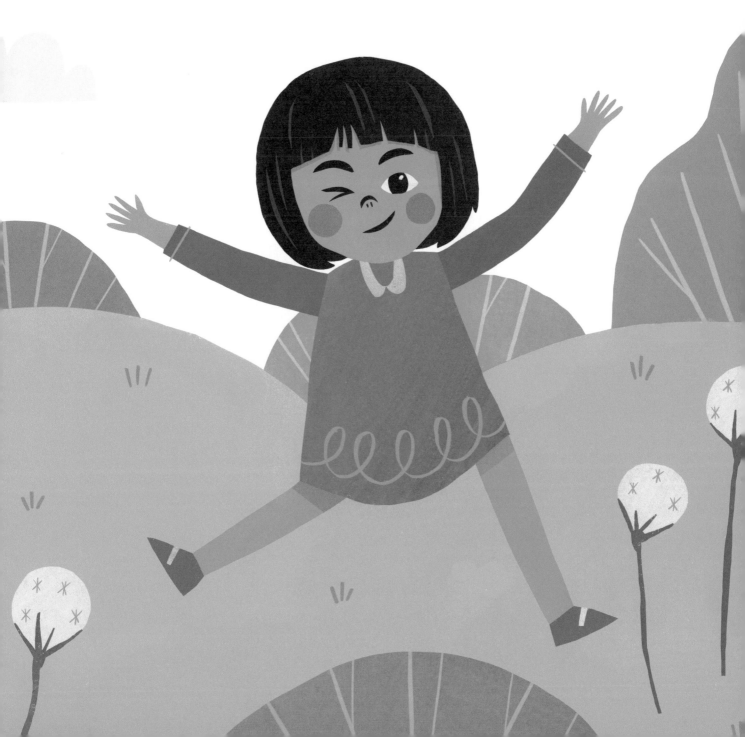

As you lie on your back,
The **trees** watch over you,
The **sunshine** warms you,
The **grass** cradles you.

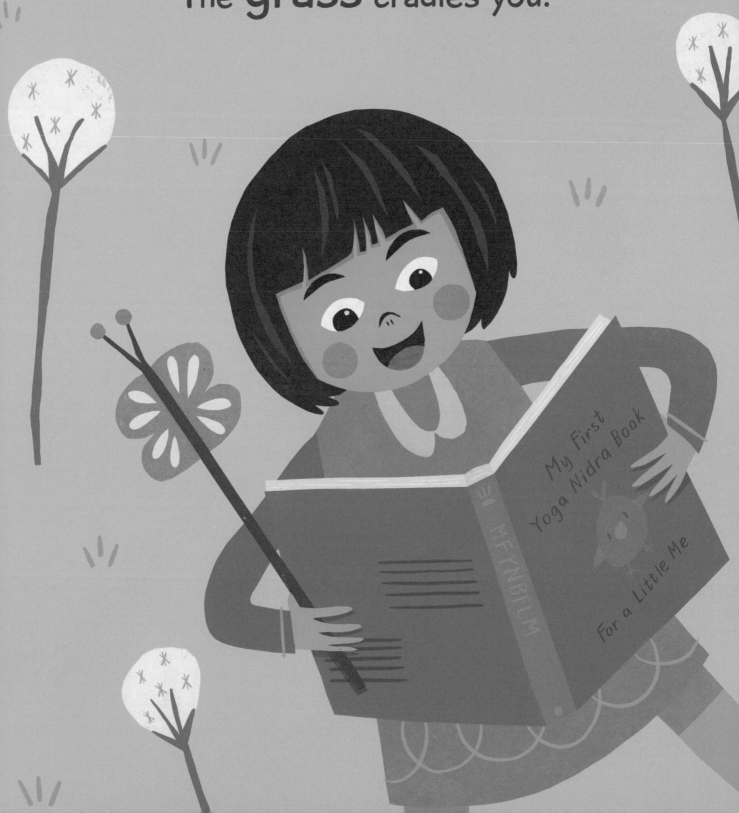

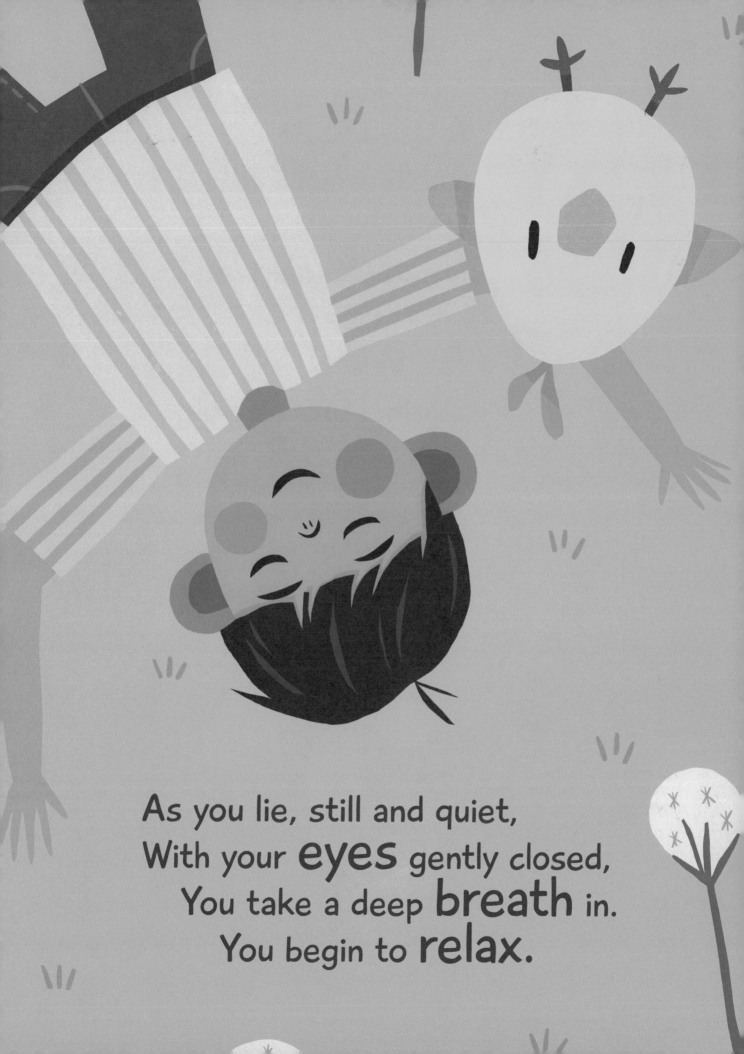

As you lie, still and quiet,
With your **eyes** gently closed,
You take a deep **breath** in.
You begin to **relax**.

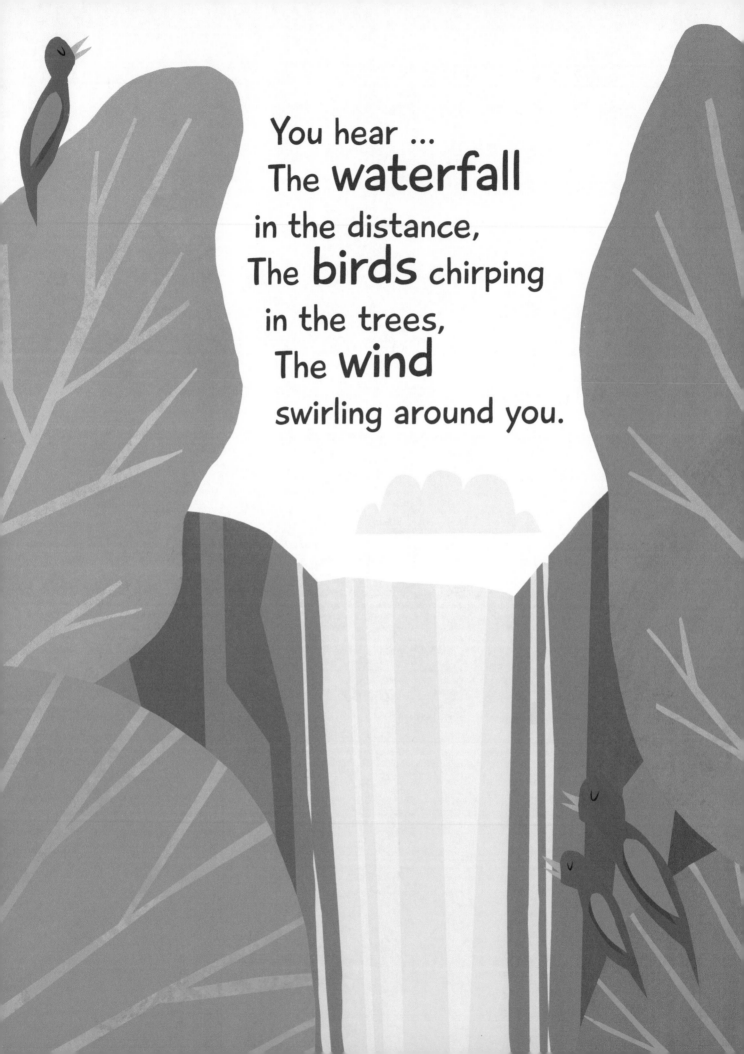

You hear ...
The **waterfall**
in the distance,
The **birds** chirping
in the trees,
The **wind**
swirling around you.

A butterfly arrives
and softly hovers over you.
The butterfly signals
the start of the journey.
The butterfly moves from
one body part to the next.
Become aware of each body part
as it is named.

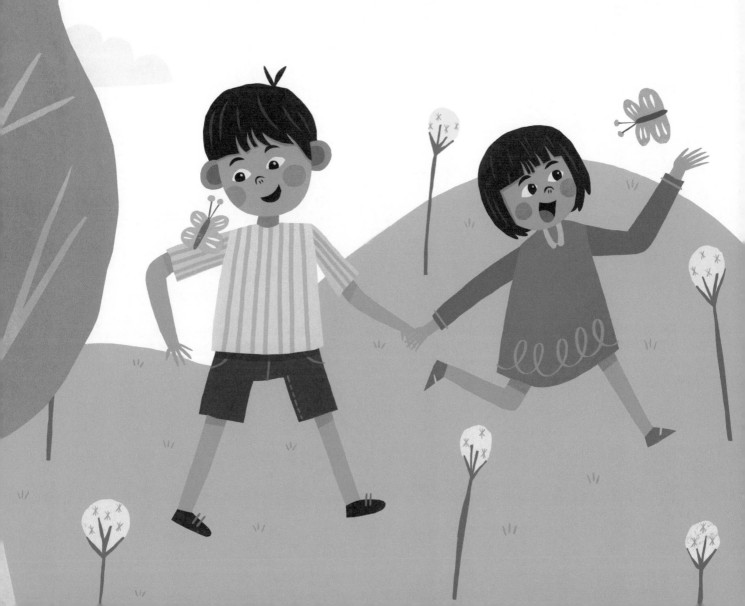

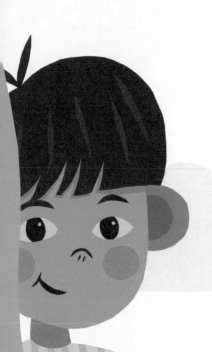

Bring awareness to the right side of the body.
Hand and fingers.
Arm and shoulder.
Waist.
Hip.
Leg.

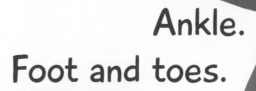

Ankle.
Foot and toes.

Bring awareness to the
left side of the body.
Hand and fingers.
Arm and shoulder.
Waist.

Hip.
Leg.
Ankle.
Foot and toes.

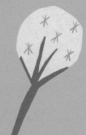

Bring awareness to
the top of the head.
Forehead.
Eyes.
Nose.
Ears.
Cheeks.
Lips.
Chin.
Neck.
Chest.
Belly.
Back.
The whole spine.

Become aware of
The whole body.
The whole body.
The whole body.

The butterfly hovers over the chest and belly.
The butterfly moves up with every breath in.
The butterfly moves down with every breath out.
Silently count each breath.

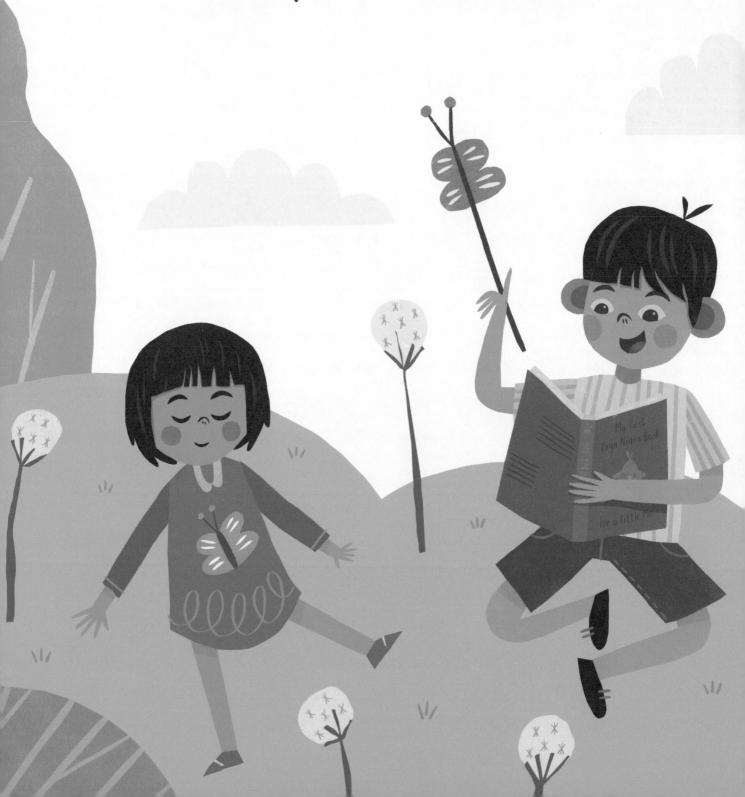

Breathe in nine,
Breathe out nine.

Breathe in eight,
Breathe out eight.

Count down seven,
six,
five,
four,
three,
two,
one.

The butterfly whispers a goodbye
and flies into the distance
With the **wind**,
With the **birds**,
Toward the
waterfall.

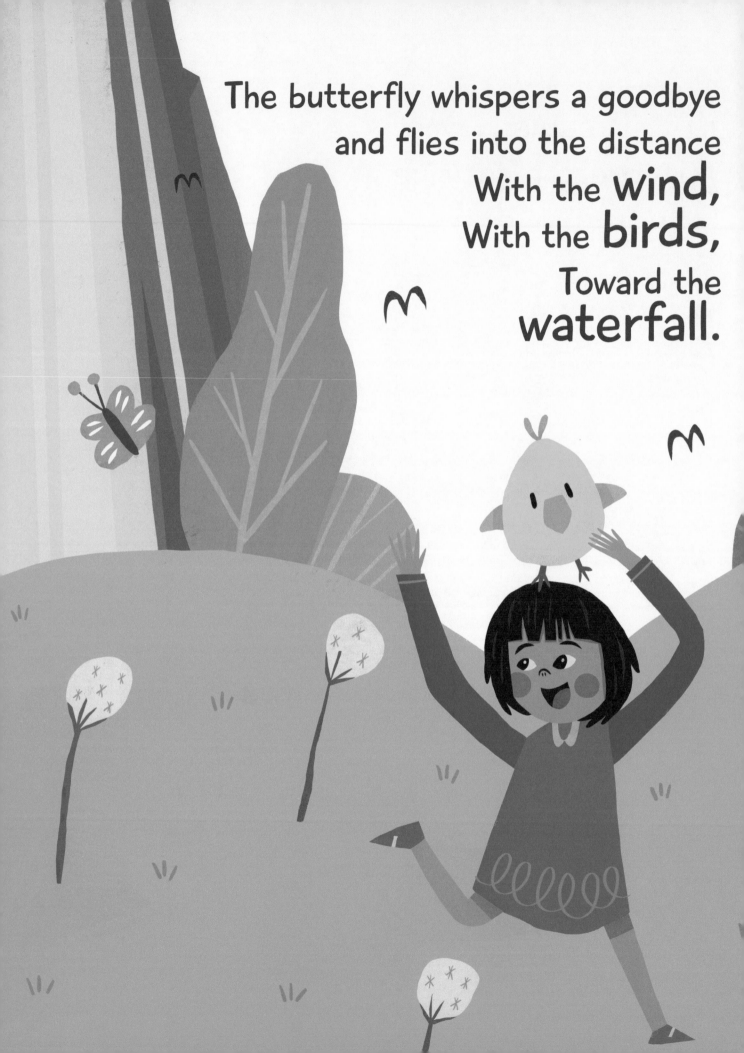

You hear ...
The **waterfall** in the distance,
The **birds** chirping in the trees,
The **wind** swirling around you.

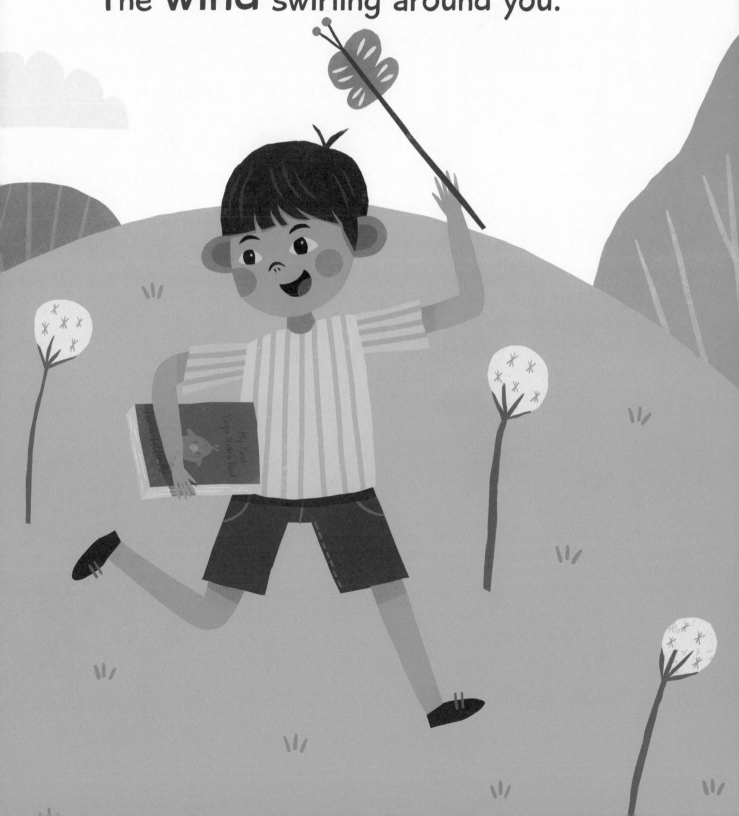

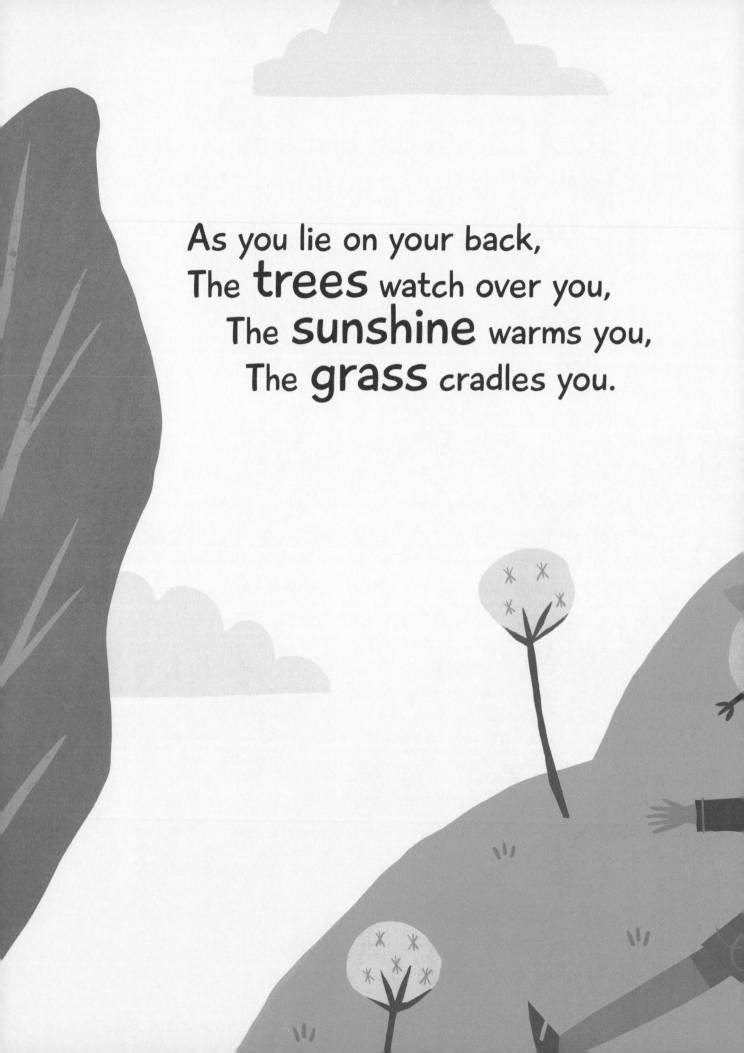

As you lie on your back,
The **trees** watch over you,
The **sunshine** warms you,
The **grass** cradles you.

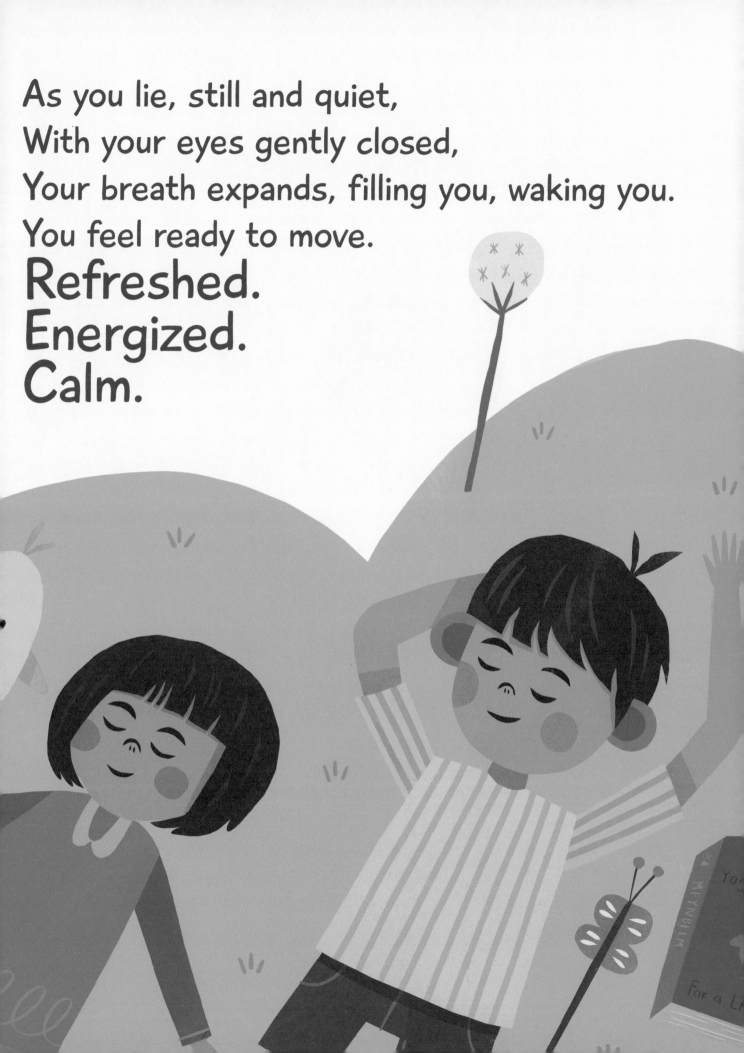

As you lie, still and quiet,
With your eyes gently closed,
Your breath expands, filling you, waking you.
You feel ready to move.
Refreshed.
Energized.
Calm.

Yoga Nidra.
A journey of the **body**.
A journey of the **breath**.
A journey.

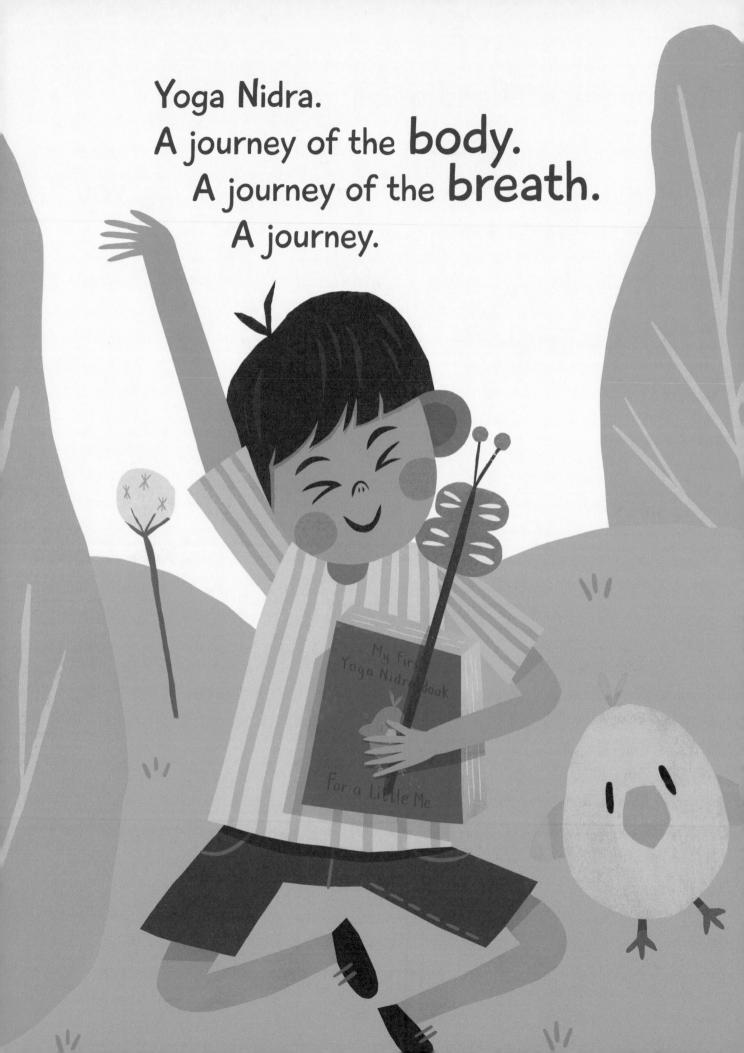

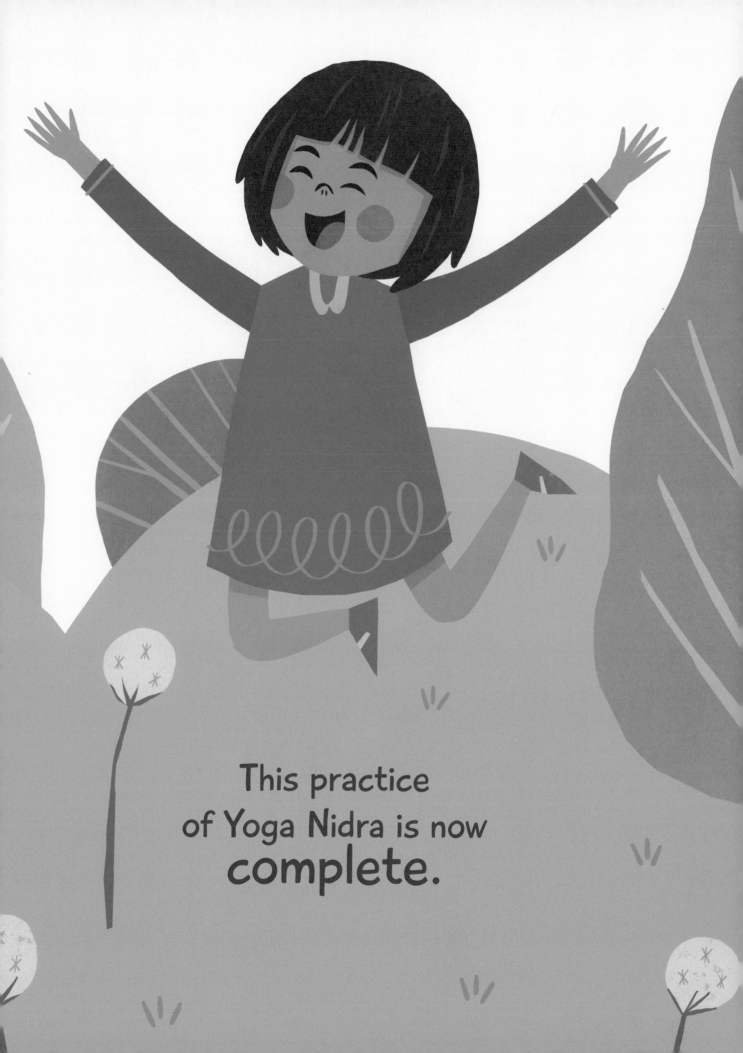

This practice
of Yoga Nidra is now
complete.

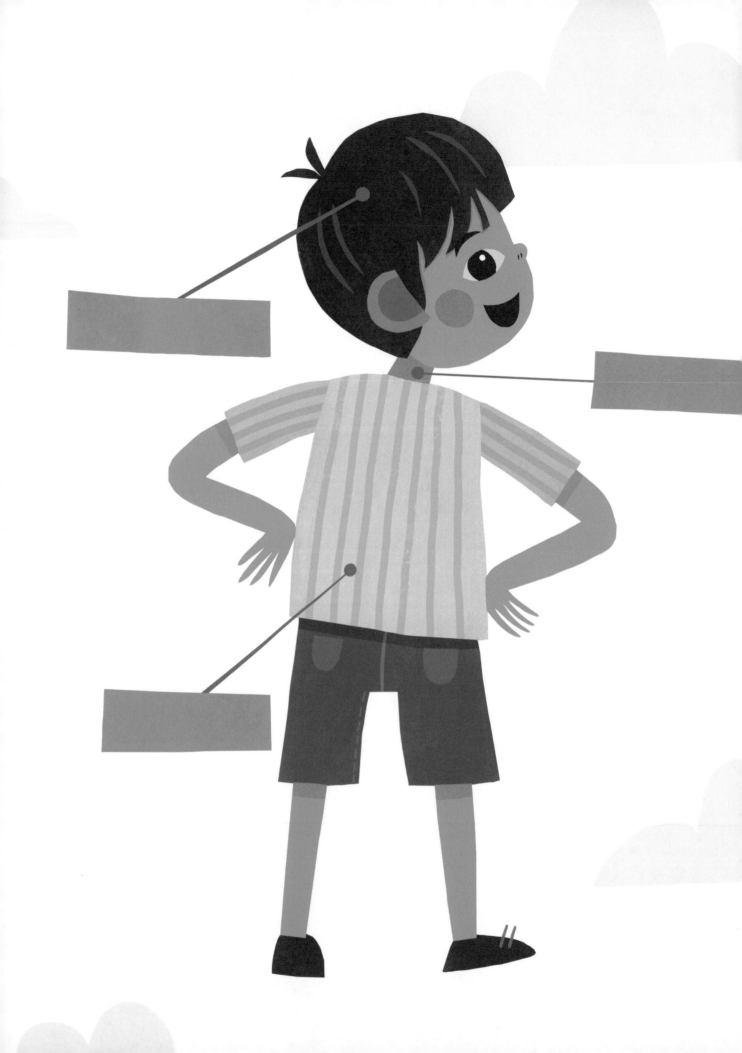

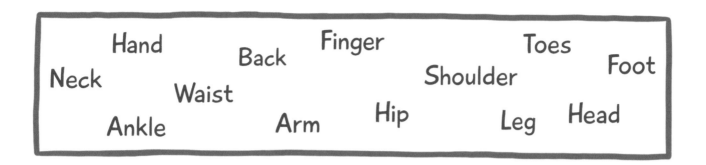

Neck Hand Back Finger Shoulder Toes Foot Waist Hip Leg Head Ankle Arm

Write the body parts in the correct box.

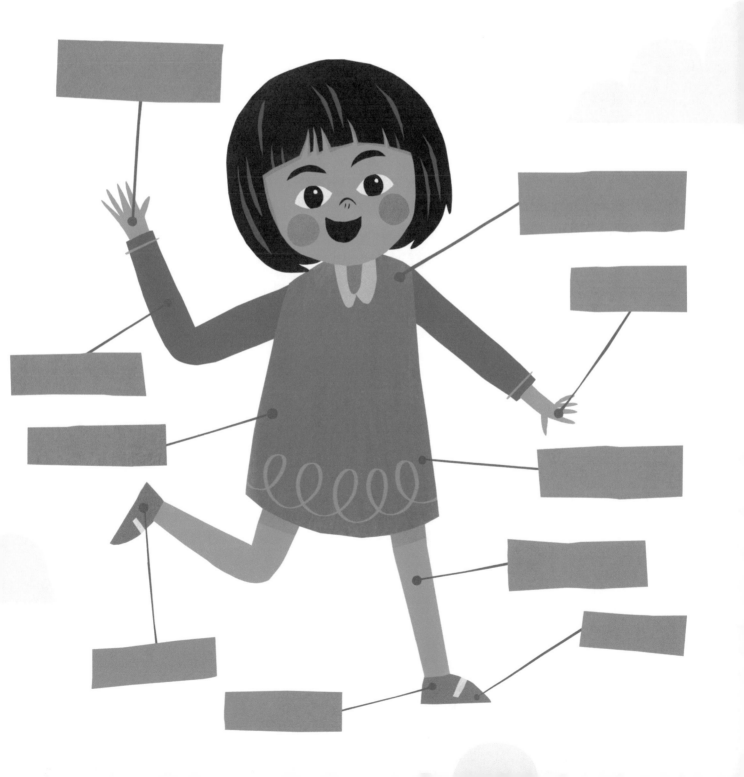

A Note to Parents and Teachers

Yoga Nidra is an ancient relaxation and meditation technique derived from the traditions of yoga. During the practice your attention moves from external sensory stimulations to the body, the breath, and eventually to the deeper aspects of the mind. This state, traditionally referred to as *pratyahara*, is experienced as relaxation with awareness. Yoga Nidra promotes physical, emotional, and mental relaxation greater than sleep itself. The practice facilitates the release of deeply held tensions as we gain access to our subconscious and unconscious mind, eventually allowing a state of homeostasis where the body can tap into its natural resources for health, healing, and wellness. A regular practice of Yoga Nidra provides several benefits, including improved energy, focus, memory, attention, and mood, more restful sleep, and reduced stress, anxiety, and pain.

The *Yoga Nidra* book is designed to introduce young readers to the practice and benefits of Yoga Nidra. The book is creatively worded to follow a traditional style of Yoga Nidra while catering to a younger audience. As they read the book, they begin to visualize and embody the practice.

For preschool and kindergarten children, it is recommended that an adult guides or reads along. For a more traditional experience, children may lie on their backs or sit with their eyes closed and have the book read to them.

Meet The Authors

Sunita Kumar, MD was born and raised in India. She moved to the United States in 1993 where she completed her residency training in psychiatry and fellowship training in geriatric psychiatry. She soon found a passion for Satyananda Yoga and Satyananda Yoga Nidra® at the Atma Center in Cleveland, Ohio. A practicing psychiatrist for over 20 years and a yoga and Yoga Nidra instructor, she regularly guided her patients in this form of meditation. She was inspired to write the *Yoga Nidra* book during her yoga teacher training with Cathy Prescott. The young boy and his little sister in the story represent her children, Rahul and Ria.

Cathy Prescott is a yoga therapist and educator based in Cleveland, Ohio. She conducts training programs for aspiring yoga teachers; specialty programs for yoga teachers and therapists, including Yoga Nidra facilitation; and is a mentor for the Kripalu School of Integrative Yoga Therapy. While her private practice currently focuses on the adult population, she taught yoga for babies, toddlers, and preschoolers with their caretakers for over a decade. Cathy can be reached at www.YogaWithCathy.com.

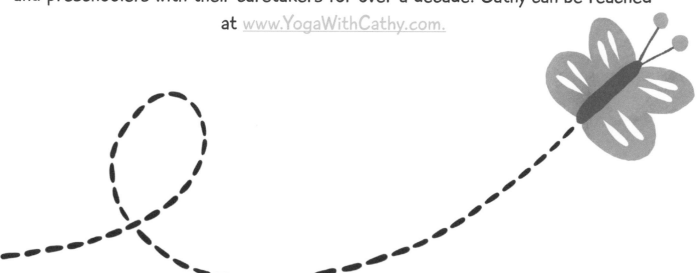

Printed in the United States
by Baker & Taylor Publisher Services